Plant-Based Soups for Everyone

Discover the Pleasures of a Plant-Based Diet with Amazing Soups Recipes

Dave Ingram

Table of contents

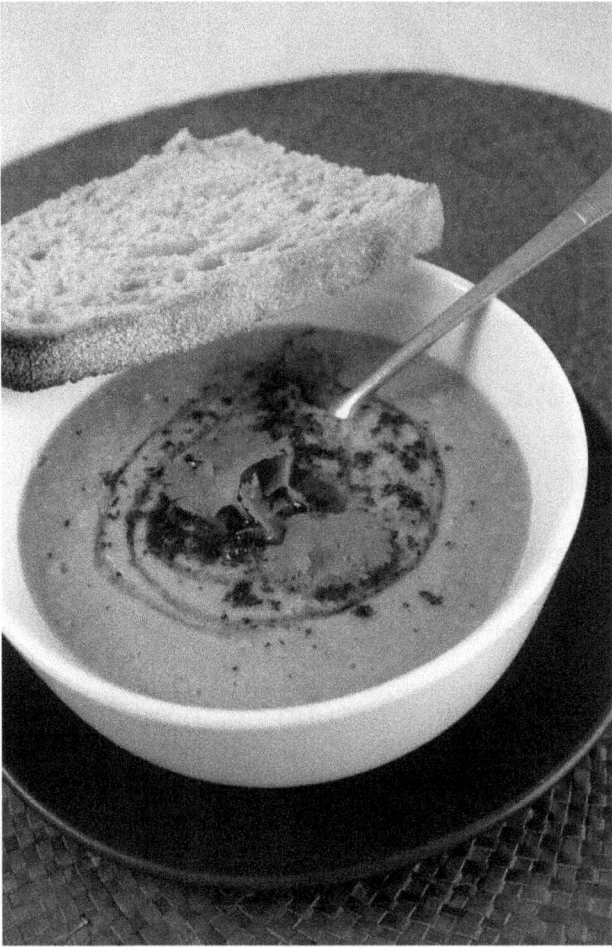

Butternut Squash Soup with Fennel

Preparation time: 15 minutes

Cook time: 25 minutes

Serves 4

Ingredients:

1 onion 2 garlic cloves

½ fennel bulb, cut into slices

1 tsbp water 2 tablespoons grated peeled fresh ginger

½ butternut squash, peeled and diced into ½-inch pieces

½ cauliflower head, cut into florets

4 to 6 cups no-sodium vegetable broth

¼ teaspoon freshly ground black pepper

Directions:

1.   Put together the onion, garlic, and fennel. Cook for 4 minutes.

2.   Cook adding the ginger and stirring, for 30 seconds.

3.   Add the butternut squash, cauliflower, and just enough vegetable broth to cover the vegetables. Simmer and cook for 15 minutes, or until the butternut squash can be easily pierced with a fork.

4.   Purée the soup until smooth.

5.   Season with pepper and serve.

Nutrition Per Serving:

calories: 91 | fat: 1g | carbs: 21g | protein: 4g | fiber: 6g

Red Lentil Stew

Preparation time: 10 minutes

Cook time: 30 minutes

Serves 8

Ingredients:

2 cups dried red lentils (masoor dal) 1 tablespoon yellow curry powder

1 teaspoon whole mustard seeds 1 teaspoon ground coriander

1 teaspoon ground cumin

8 cups water, plus 3 tablespoons and more as needed 1 large yellow onion, finely diced

6 garlic cloves, minced

1 tablespoon minced peeled fresh ginger 1 celery stalk, finely chopped

2 green chiles, minced (and seeded if you want less heat) 1 (15-ounce /425-g) can diced tomatoes

Fresh cilantro, for garnish

Directions:

1.   Place the lentils in a fine-mesh sieve. Sift through them to look for stones or other debris. Rinse under cold water for a few minutes.

2.   In a small dish, combine the curry powder, mustard seeds, coriander, and cumin. Set aside.

3.   Put together lentils and 8 cups of water. Bring to a boil. Turn the heat to medium-low, partially cover the pot, and cook for 20 minutes. The lentils should be very tender.

4.   While the lentils cook, make the tadka or tempered spices. Mix the onion, garlic, ginger, celery, and green chiles. Cook for 5 minutes, adding water, 1 tablespoon of at a time, to prevent burning. The onion should be deeply browned and soft.

5.   Spread the mixture out in the pan so that there is a small well or opening in the center. Pour the spices into the well and add 2 tablespoons of water. Cook for 1 minute, stirring continuously, slowly mixing the spices into the cooked vegetables.

6.   Carefully add the tomatoes and stir to combine. Cook over medium-low heat for 7 minutes, stirring frequently.

7.   Add the tadka to the cooked lentils, stir well, and cook for 5 minutes over medium heat. Serve immediately, garnished with cilantro, or refrigerate and serve the following day. Dal gets more flavorful with a day or two of resting in the refrigerator.

Nutrition Per Serving:

calories: 206 | fat: 1g | carbs: 37g | protein: 13g | fiber: 7g

Roasted Red Pepper and Squash Soup

Preparation time: 10 minutes

Cook time: 40 to 50 minutes

Makes 6 bowls

Ingredients:

1 small butternut squash 1 tablespoon olive oil

1 teaspoon sea salt 2 red bell peppers 1 yellow onion

1 head garlic

2 cups water, or vegetable broth Zest and juice of 1 lime

1 to 2 tablespoons tahini Pinch cayenne pepper

½ teaspoon ground coriander

½ teaspoon ground cumin Toasted squash seeds (optional)

Directions:

1.   Heat the oven to 180°

2.   Prepare the squash for roasting by cutting it in half lengthwise, scooping out the seeds. Rub a small amount

of oil over the flesh and skin, rub with a bit of sea salt and put the halves skin- side down in a large baking dish. Put it in the oven while you prepare the rest of the vegetables.

3.   Prepare the peppers the same way, except they do not need to be poked. Slice the onion in half and rub oil on the exposed faces.

4.   Add peppers, onion, and garlic, and roast for another 20 minutes. Optionally, you can toast the squash seeds by putting them in the oven in a separate baking dish 10 to 15 minutes before the vegetables are finished. Keep a close eye on them.

5.   When cooked, let them cool before handling them. The squash will be very soft when poked with a fork.

6.   Scoop into a large pot (if you have an immersion blender) or into a blender. Chop the pepper roughly, remove the onion skin and chop the onion roughly, and squeeze the garlic cloves out of the head, all into the pot or blender. Add the water, the lime zest and juice, and the tahini. Purée the soup, adding more water if you like, to your desired consistency.

7.   Season with salt, cayenne, coriander, and cumin. Serve garnished with toasted squash seeds (if using).

Nutrition Per Serving (1 bowl):

calories: 156 | fat: 10g | carbs: 6g | protein: 4g | fiber: 5g

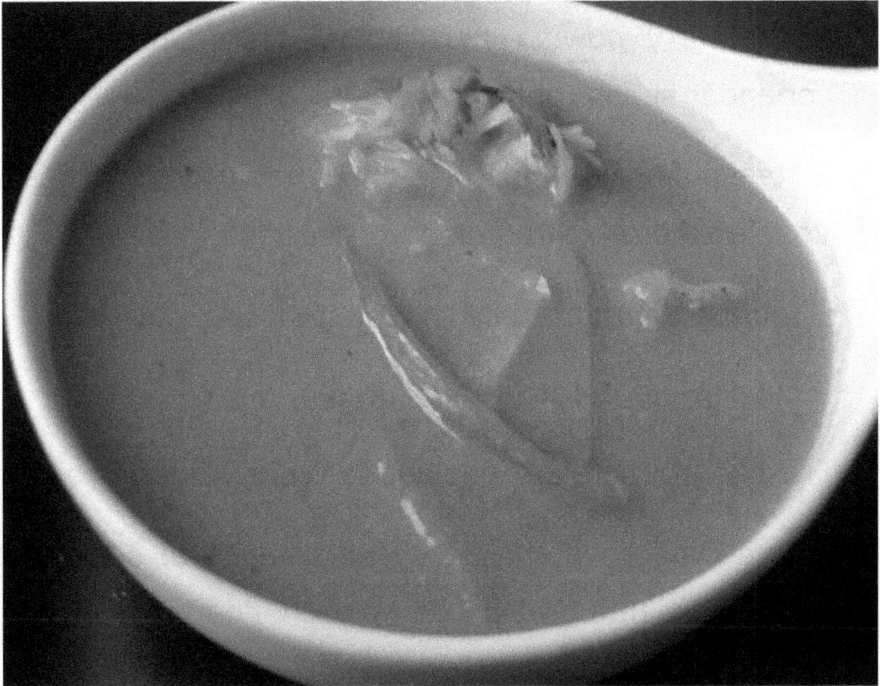

Indian Red Split Lentil Soup

Preparation time: 5 minutes

Cook time: 50 minutes

Makes 4 bowls

Ingredients:

1 cup lentils 3 cups water

1 tsp curry powder plus 1 tablespoon, divided, or 5 coriander seeds (optional)

1 teaspoon coconut oil, or 1 tablespoon water or vegetable broth 1 red onion, diced

1 tablespoon minced fresh ginger

3 cups sweet potato 1 cup zucchini

Freshly ground black pepper, to taste Sea salt, to taste

3 to 4 cups vegetable stock, or water 1 to 2 teaspoons toasted sesame oil 1 bunch spinach, chopped

Toasted sesame seeds

Directions:

1.   Boil the lentils and simmer for 10 minutes, until the lentils are soft.

2.   Add the coconut oil and sauté the onion and ginger until soft, about 5 minutes. Add the sweet potato and leave it on the heat for about 10 minutes to soften slightly, then add the zucchini and cook until it starts to look shiny about 5 minutes. Add the remaining 1 tablespoon curry powder, pepper, and salt, and stir the vegetables to coat.

3.   Add the vegetable stock, bring to a boil, then turn down to simmer and cover. Let the vegetables slowly cook for 20 to 30 minutes or until the sweet potato is tender.

4.   Add the fully cooked lentils to the soup. Add another pinch of salt, the toasted sesame oil, and the spinach. Stir, allowing the spinach to wilt before removing the pot from the heat.

5.   Serve garnished with toasted sesame seeds.

Nutrition Per Serving (1 bowl):

calories: 319 | fat: 18g | carbs: 5g | protein: 16g | fiber: 10g

Split Pea Soup with Tomatoes

Preparation time: 15 minutes

Cook time: 60 to 75 minutes

Makes 6 bowls

Ingredients:

¼ glass white wine, or vegetable stock, or water 1 onion, chopped

1 to 2 garlic cloves, 1 cup peas

3 bay (leaves)

1 tbsp thyme 1 tbsp oregano

3 to 4 cups water or salt-free vegetable stock

1 large carrot or zucchini, chopped (optional)

1 tablespoon miso, or tamari, or ¼ teaspoon sea salt Pinch freshly ground black pepper

2 tablespoons nutritional yeast (optional)

¼ cup sun-dried tomatoes, or olives, chopped

¼ cup cherry tomatoes, chopped 2 tablespoons chopped scallions

Directions:

1.   Put together onion, wine. Add garlic and stir for 5 minutes. Add the peas and the bay leaves, thyme, and oregano. Pour in the water and take it to boil.

2.   Leave the peas to cook.

3.   Add the carrot (if using) about 20 minutes before you finish cooking the soup. This will allow it to soften but not overcook.

4.   Once the peas are soft, take the bay leaves out and purée the soup in the blender or with an immersion blender. Return to the pot.

5.   Stir in the miso, pepper, and nutritional yeast (if using), and then add the sun-dried tomatoes.

6.   Serve topped with cherry tomatoes and some scallions.

Nutrition Per Serving (1 bowl)

calories: 183 | fat: 11g | carbs: 3g | protein: 12g | fiber: 12g

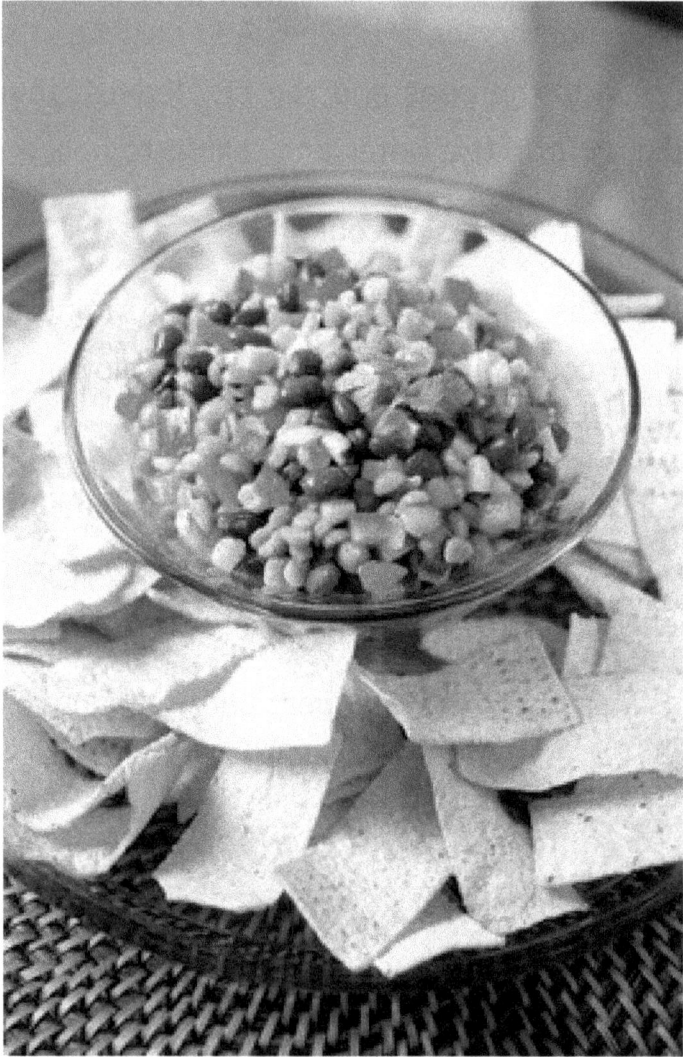

Cream of Broccoli Soup

Preparation time: 10 minutes

Cook time: 25 minutes

Serves 6

Ingredients:

4 leeks 1 tsp thyme

5 cups broccoli florets 4½ cups vegetable stock, plus more as needed

1 tbsp nutritional yeast (optional) Salt and black pepper

Directions:

1.   Sauté the leeks for 10 minutes. Add the thyme, broccoli, vegetable stock, and nutritional yeast. Leti t cook until the broccoli is tender, about 10 minutes.

2.   Purée the soup using an immersion blender.

Red Lentil Soup with Farro

Cook time: 32 minutes

Servings: 4

Ingredients:

½ cup red lentils

½ cup quick-cook farro

1 cup kale, stemmed, chopped 1 cup carrots, grated

2 tablespoons olive oil 5 cups vegetable broth 1 small onion, grated

1 small zucchini, grated 1 ½ teaspoon turmeric

½ teaspoon cumin

¼ teaspoon pepper 1 ½ teaspoons salt

For breadcrumbs:

Eight slices French baguette, cubed Olive oil

One garlic clove, minced Salt, to taste

Directions:

1.   Sauté onion, carrots, and zucchini in olive oil over medium heat for 2 minutes. Stir in the turmeric, cumin, pepper, and salt, then cook for 3 minutes.

2.   Bring it to a boil adding the chicken broth. Add lentils and farro and cook for about 20 minutes over low heat.

3.   In the meantime, pulse bread and garlic in a food processor until done. Add olive oil and salt

— Bake for 7 minutes.

4.   Once the lentil soup has been cooked for 15 minutes, add kale and cook for 5 minutes. Serve topped with breadcrumbs.

Moroccan Pumpkin Soup

Cook time: 50 minutes

Servings: 4-6

Ingredients:

3 lbs pumpkin, peeled, seeded, chopped 2 carrots, roughly chopped

1/3 cup split peas

3 tablespoons olive oil

3 tablespoons white miso paste 1 onion, diced

1 cinnamon stick

1 chili, finely chopped 1 garlic, finely chopped

1 small ginger, thinly sliced 1 ½ teaspoon cumin seeds

Directions:

1.   Cook garlic, onions, and salt in olive oil over low heat for 3 minutes. Add all the spices and sauté until fragrant.

2.   Stir in pumpkin, carrots, and peas. Bring to a boil. Simmer for extra 30 minutes. Remove and discard the cinnamon stick.

3.   Puree the soup until smooth, then let cool. Stir in the miso paste and serve just after that.

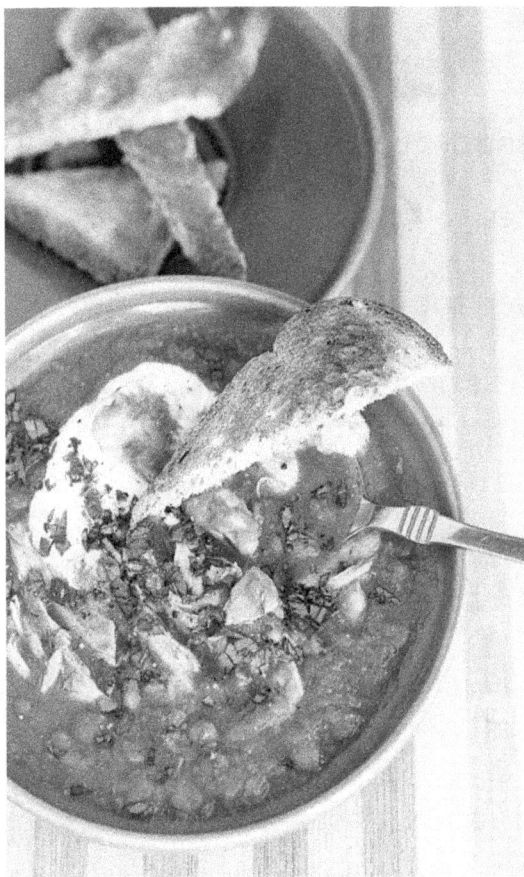

Mexican Chickpea and Tomatillos Pozole

Cook time: 20 minutes

Servings: 2-4

Ingredients:

1 ½ cups chickpeas, cooked

10 tomatillos, peeled, washed 2 cups of water

1 cup cilantro, chopped 4 garlic cloves

¼ onion, sliced

1 whole serrano chile

1 teaspoon salt, or to taste

Directions:

1.   Add tomatillos, cilantro, onion, garlic, and water into a large pot. Cook, covered until tomatillos are very soft.

2.   Add salt to taste and puree using an immersion blender; blend the vegetables until adequately combined. Stir in the chickpeas and serrano chile.

3. Enjoy with your desired toppings.

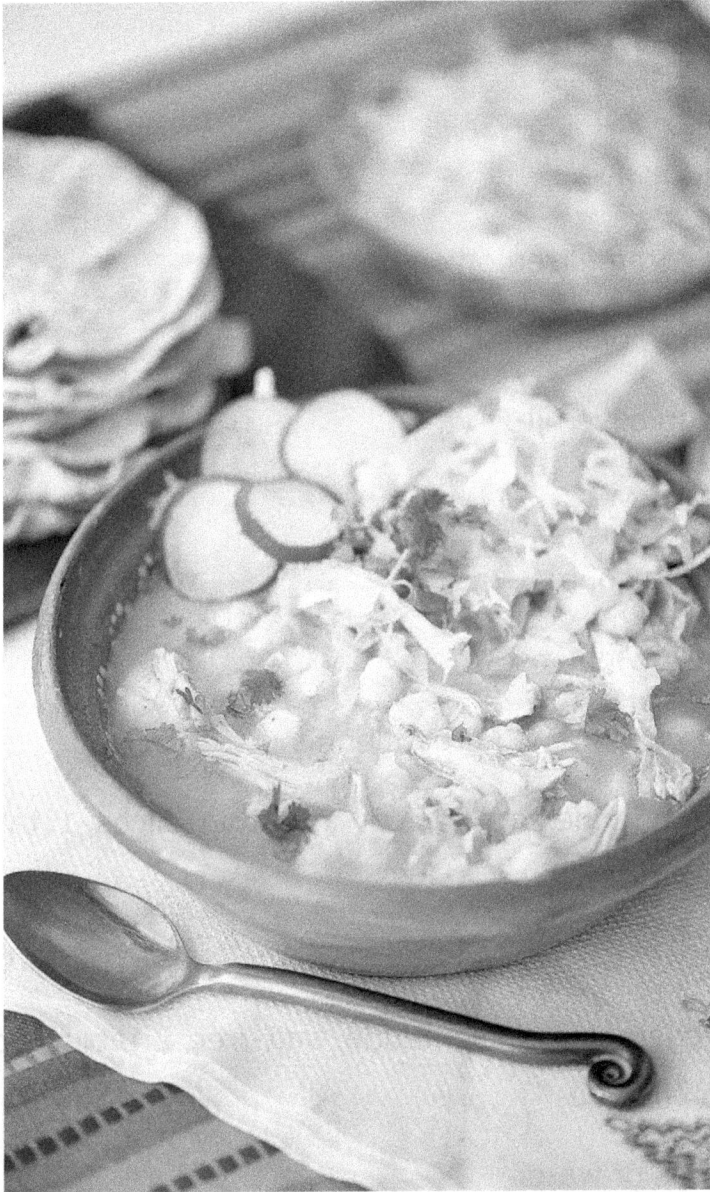

Vegan French Onion Soup

Cook time: 115 minutes

Servings: 2-4

Ingredients:

For caramelized onions:

4 white onions

¼ cup olive oil

For the soup:

4 yellow onions

1 ½ cups French green lentils

1 cup fennel stalks, cut into thin slices 1 tablespoon tarragon leaves

1 bay leaf

3 vegetable bouillon cube, salt-free 2 tablespoons + ¼ cup olive oil

8 cups of water

6 tablespoons dry white wine 1 tablespoon Sherry vinegar

1 tablespoon fresh lemon juice

½ teaspoon black pepper

1   tablespoon + 1 teaspoon salt 2 tablespoons fresh thyme

2   garlic cloves, minced

Directions:

For the onions:

1.   Slice onions into thin half circles. Cook on medium heat, infrequently stirring, for 20 minutes (without oil).

2.   Pour in ¼ cup olive oil. Scrape the bottom of the pan using a wooden spatula. Stir and reduce the heat to medium-low. Cook for 20 minutes, stirring infrequently. Set aside.

For the soup:

1.   Deglaze a pan by scraping the bottom of the pan with a wooden spatula. Let rest for 10 minutes.

2. Pour in 2 more tablespoons of wine, deglaze and cook for 10 minutes. Add an extra tablespoon of wine, deglaze and turn the heat offseason with salt.

3. Combine lentils, water, bay leaf, and two sprigs of thyme in a large pot. Cook until it boils. Simmer on medium-low heat for extra 20 minutes.

4. Meanwhile, sauté sliced fennel stalks and garlic in olive oil over medium-low heat until garlic is fragrant.

5. Add tarragon, bouillon cubes, and two tablespoons of thyme. Mash the bouillon. Stir the ingredients, then add one tablespoon of wine. Cook the stalks, frequently stirring until they turn golden. Pour in the remaining wine.

6. Pour the sautéed fennel stalk mixture and the caramelized onions into the cooked lentils. Mix in 2 tablespoons water, sherry vinegar, lemon juice, pepper, and salt, then cook for some minutes before serving.

Mexican Lentil Soup

Total time: 55 minutes

Ingredients:

2 tbsp extra-virgin olive oil 2 carrots

1 onion 1 red bell pepper 2 celery stalks

1 tbsp of cumin

3 cloves of garlic (minced)

3 cups of green lentils 2 cups of tomatoes (diced), and the juice

8 cups of vegetable broth

½ tsp of salt

2 cans of green chile (diced)

¼ tsp paprika 1 tsp oregano

1 avocado 1 cilantro

Hot sauce (optional and for serving)

Directions:

1.   Cook the carrots, onion, bell pepper, and celery until softened, 5 minutes. Season with cumin, garlic, pepper, and cook for another minute.

2.   Mix in the lentils, tomatoes, broth, salt, and green chilies. Bring to a boil, cover the lid, and simmer until the lentils soften 10 to 15 minutes.

3.   Season with salt and pepper.

4.   Top with the avocado, cilantro, and hot sauce.

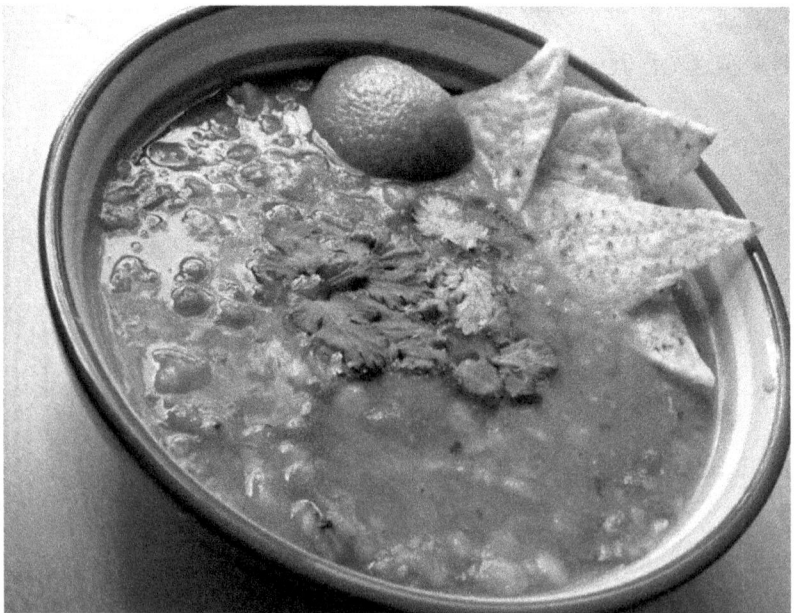

Lovely Parsnip & Split Pea Soup

Total time: 5 hours 10 minutes

Ingredients:

1 tablespoon of olive oil

3 parsnips 2 large carrots, peeled and chopped

1 medium-sized white onion, peeled and diced 1 1/2 teaspoon of minced garlic

2 1/4 cups of dried green split peas, rinsed 1 teaspoon of salt

1/2 teaspoon of ground black pepper 1 teaspoon of dried thyme

2 bay leaves

6 cups broth 1 tsp of liquid smoke

Directions:

1.   Place a   medium-sized   non-stick skilletpan   over an   average pressure of heat, add the oil and let it heat.

2.   Add the parsnip, carrot, onion, garlic and let it cook for 5 minutes or until it is heated.

3.   Transfer this mixture into a 6-quart slow cooker and add the remaining ingredients.

4.   Stir until mixes properly and cover the top.

5.   Plug in the slow cooker; adjust the cooking time to 5 hours and let it cook on the high heat setting or until the peas and vegetables get soft.

6.   When done, remove the bay leaf from the soup and blend it with a submersion blender or until the soup reaches your desired state.

7.   Add the seasoning and serve.

Tomato Artichoke Soup

Preparation Time: 5 minutes

Cooking Time: 35 minutes

Servings: 4

Ingredients:

1 can artichoke 1 can tomatoes 3 cups vegetable broth

1 small onion, chopped

2 cloves garlic, crushed 1 tbsp. pesto

Black pepper, to taste

Directions:

1.   Combine all ingredients in the slow cooker.

2.   Cook on high for 4-5 hours.

3.   Blend the soup in batches, then put it back in the slow cooker. Season with pepper and salt, then serve.

Nutrition: Calories: 1487 kcal Protein: 3.98 g Fat: 167.42 g Carbohydrates:8.2 g

Garlicky Cauliflower and Potato Soup

Preparation time: 20 minutes

Cook time: 30 minutes

Serves 6

Ingredients:

8 garlic cloves, peeled

1 cauliflower head

2 potatoes 1 yellow onion, coarsely chopped

1 celery stalk, coarsely chopped

1 tbsp water, plus more as needed 6 cups no-sodium vegetable broth

2 thyme sprigs

2 teaspoons paprika

¼ teaspoon freshly ground black pepper

1 tablespoon chopped fresh rosemary leaves

Directions:

1.	Heat the oven to 235ºC. Line a baking sheet with parchment paper.

2.	Wrap the garlic cloves in aluminum foil or place them in a garlic roaster.

3.	Evenly spread the cauliflower and potatoes on the prepared baking sheet.

4.	Roast unitl cauliflower is lightly browned.

5.	Put together onion and celery. Sauté for 4 to 5 minutes, adding water, 1 tablespoon at a time, to prevent burning, until the onion starts to brown.

6.	Bring soup to a simmer.

7.	Add the roasted vegetables and garlic, thyme, paprika, and pepper. Cook for 10 minutes.

8.	Remove and discard the thyme. Purée the soup until smooth.

9.	Stir in the rosemary.

Moroccan Chickpea Stew

Preparation time: 20 minutes

Cook time: 30 minutes

Serves 4

Ingredients:

1 tbsp Hungarian paprika 1 tsp smoked paprika

1 tsp cumin 1 tsp onion powder

1 large yellow onion, coarsely chopped 4 garlic cloves, diced

1 tbsp water 2 carrots, diced

1 tablespoon pure maple syrup

1 (28-ounce / 794-g) can crushed tomatoes

½ cup packed chopped fresh cilantro

1 can chickpeas,

1 dark red kidney beans Juice of ½ lime

Directions:

1.   In a small bowl, stir together the Hungarian paprika, smoked paprika, cumin, and onion powder. Set aside.

2.   Put together onion, garlic, and 1 tablespoon of water. Turn the heat to medium-low. Cook for at least 10 minutes, stirring occasionally.

3.   Stir in the carrots. Turn the heat to high.

4.   Stir in the paprika mixture and cook for 30 seconds, stirring continuously to prevent burning. Cook 30 seconds more, adding the syrup and stirring.

5.   Carefully pour in the tomatoes with their juices. To avoid splatter, pour the tomatoes onto a spoon and not directly into the hot pot. Bring to a simmer, stirring, turn the heat to low, cover the pot, and cook for 10 minutes.

6.   Stir in the cilantro, chickpeas, and kidney beans.

7.   Sprinkle with lime juice before serving.

NutritionPer Serving

calories: 331 | fat: 3g | carbs: 65g | protein: 17g | fiber: 15g

Acorn Squash Curry Soup

Preparation time: 20 minutes

Cook time: 1 hour

Serves 6

Ingredients:

1 acorn squash

1 onion, chopped 2 garlic cloves

2 celery stalks, coarsely chopped

1 tbsp water 2 tablespoons whole wheat flour

2 cups no-sodium vegetable broth

1 teaspoon curry powder, plus more for seasoning

½ teaspoon dill

⅛ teaspoon cayenne pepper

1 (14-ounce / 397-g) can full-fat coconut milk Chopped scallions, green parts only, for serving

Directions:

1. Heat the oven to 180ºC.

2. Place the squash halves, cut-side down, in a 9-by-13- inch baking dish, and add enough water to come up about 1 inch all around.

3. Bake for 30 to 45 minutes, or until the squash is easily pierced with a fork.

4. Put together onion, garlic, and celery. Sauté for 2 to 3 minutes.

5. Add the vegetable broth, roasted squash, curry powder, dill, and cayenne pepper. Bring the mixture to a boil. Cook for 10 minutes.

6. Pour in the coconut milk. Blend the soup until smooth. Serve immediately.

7. Top with scallions and a sprinkle of curry powder.

Nutrition Per Serving:

calories: 169 | fat: 13g | carbs: 14g | protein: 2g | fiber: 2g

Creamy Tomato and Carrot Soup

Preparation time: 10 minutes

Cook time: 35 minutes

Serves 4

Ingredients:

2 carrots, coarsely chopped

½ cup water, plus 1 tablespoon and more as needed 1 yellow onion, coarsely chopped

2 to 4 garlic cloves, coarsely chopped

1 (6-ounce / 170-g) can tomato paste 1 tablespoon Hungarian paprika

1 (28-ounce / 794-g) can diced tomatoes

1 (14-ounce / 397-g) can full-fat coconut milk 1 teaspoon dried thyme

No-sodium vegetable broth or water for thinning (optional)

Directions:

1.   Cook the carrots for 10 minutes, or until the carrots can be easily pierced with a fork. Add more water, ¼ cup at a time, if the water evaporates while cooking. Drain and transfer the cooked carrots to a bowl. Set aside.

2.   Place the same pot over medium-low heat and combine the onion and garlic. Sauté for 5 to 7 minutes, adding water, 1 tablespoon at a time, to prevent burning, until the onion is fully browned.

3.   Turn the heat to medium-high. Add the tomato paste and paprika.

4.   Add the diced tomatoes, coconut milk, thyme, and cooked carrots. Bring the liquid to a simmer. Cook for 10 minutes, stirring occasionally.

5.   Blend the soup until smooth. Alternatively, transfer the soup to a standard blender, working in batches as needed, and blend until smooth.

6.   Add vegetable broth or water to thin as needed.

Nutrition Per Serving:

calories: 292 | fat: 19g | carbs: 28g | protein: 6g | fiber: 7g

Roasted Eggplant and Lentil Stew

Preparation time: 20 minutes

Cook time: 1 hour

Serves 8

Ingredients:

1 large eggplant

4 carrots, coarsely chopped

4 cups no-sodium vegetable broth 1 cup dried brown or green lentils 1 large yellow onion, diced

1 bunch chopped callions 3 garlic cloves, diced

1 tablespoon water, plus more as needed

1 (14-ounce / 397-g) can full-fat coconut milk 1 tablespoon red miso paste

1 tablespoon low-sodium soy sauce

1 (28-ounce / 794-g) can diced tomatoes 4 teaspoons ground cumin

1 teaspoon adobo chili powder or smoked paprika

1 celery stalk, coarsely chopped fresh cilantro leaves, for serving

Directions:

1.   Heat the oven to 180ºC.

2.   Halve the eggplant lengthwise and place it on a baking sheet, flesh- side up. Spread the carrots around the eggplant on the same baking sheet.

3.   Let it roast until the eggplant and carrots are lightly browned or caramel-colored, and the carrots are fork-tender.

4.   Set the carrots aside. Let the eggplant cool before handling it.

5.   Bring the vegetable broth to a boil. Add the lentils. Cover the pot and cook for 20 to 30 minutes, or until the lentils are soft yet retain their shape.

6.   While the lentils cook in a small sauté pan or skillet over medium heat, cook the onion, white parts of the scallion, and garlic for 7 to 10 minutes.

7.   In a blender, combine the roasted eggplant and onion mixture with coconut milk, miso paste, and soy sauce. Purée for 2 to 3 minutes until smooth.

8.   Once the lentils are finished cooking, add the tomatoes, cumin, chili powder, and celery. Bring the mixture to a simmer. Pour in the eggplant sauce and add the roasted carrots. Cook until warmed to your liking.

9.   This stew is best served with a few fresh cilantro leaves and scallion greens on top.

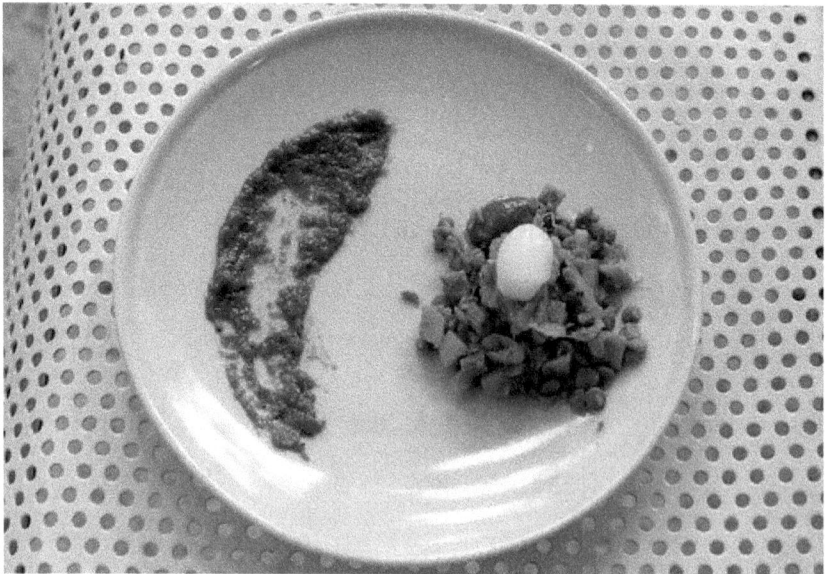

Hungarian Red Lentil Soup

Preparation time: 10 minutes

Cook time: 25 minutes

Serves 4

Ingredients:

1 onion, diced 3 garlic cloves, minced

3 cups water, plus 1 tablespoon and more as needed

4 ounces (113 g) tomato paste

2 tablespoons Hungarian paprika, plus more for seasoning 1 teaspoon ground mustard

¼ tsp black pepper

3 carrots, diced

1 celery stalk, diced

1 cup dried red lentils, rinsed

1 (14-ounce / 397-g) can light coconut milk Chopped scallions, green parts only, for serving

Directions:

1.   Combine onion and garlic. Sauté for 2 to 3 minutes.

2.   Add the tomato paste, paprika, mustard, and pepper. Cook, stirring, for 2 minutes.

3.   Add the carrots and celery. Bring the soup to a simmer and add the lentils. Cook for 10 minutes.

4.   Stir in the coconut milk and bring the mixture to a simmer, stirring continuously. Cook for 5 minutes, or until the lentils are tender.

5.   Serve topped with scallions and a sprinkle of Hungarian paprika and pepper.

Nutrition Per Serving:

calories: 309 | fat: 9g | carbs: 48g | protein: 15g | fiber: 10g

Vegetable Barley Soup

Preparation time: 10 minutes

Cook time: 25 minutes

Serves 4

Ingredients:

6 multicolored carrots, cut into 1-inch pieces

½ cup barley

1 (15-ounce /425-g) can dice tomatoes 2 garlic cloves, minced

4 cups no-sodium vegetable broth 2 cups water

4 cups fresh spinach

¼ cup chopped fresh basil leaves, plus more for garnish

2 tbsp chives

1 (15-ounce /425-g) can cannellini beans, rinsed and drained 1 tablespoon balsamic vinegar

Freshly ground black pepper, to taste

Directions:

1.	Mix the carrots, barley, tomatoes with their juices, garlic, vegetable broth, and water. Bring to a simmer. Cook until the barley is chewy and not hard.

2.	Place spinach, basil, and chives on top of the water but do not stir.

3.	Stir the pot and add the cannellini beans and vinegar. Leti t cool for 5 minutes. Garnish with chives, basil, and a pinch of pepper to serve.

Nutrition Per Serving:

calories: 261 | fat: 2g | carbs: 50g | protein: 12g | fiber: 14g

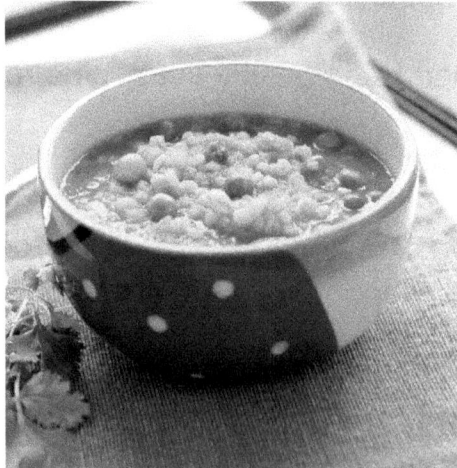

Mushroom Wild Rice Soup

Preparation time: 15 minutes

Cook time: 45 minutes

Serves 4

Ingredients:

4 cups no-sodium vegetable broth

½ cup walnuts

9 ounces (255 g) baby portabella mushrooms, coarsely chopped 4 ounces (113 g) shiitake mushrooms, coarsely chopped

1 tablespoon balsamic vinegar, plus more for drizzling 4 garlic cloves, minced

½ celery stalk, minced 3 thyme sprigs, divided

3 tablespoons whole wheat flour 4 cups unsweetened almond milk

½ cup wild rice

½ cup brown rice 1 rosemary sprig

Freshly ground black pepper, to taste

Directions:

1.   In a high-speed blender, combine the vegetable broth and walnuts. Let sit for 1 hour to soften the walnuts. You can also soak the walnuts overnight in an airtight glass container.

2.   In an 8-quart pot over medium-high heat, combine the portabella and shiitake mushrooms. Cook for 5 minutes to expel most of the liquid from the mushrooms. Pour on the vinegar and cook for 1 minute more. Turn off the heat. Transfer the mushrooms to a non-plastic bowl.

3.   Transfer ¼ cup of the mushroom mixture to the blender with the vegetable broth and walnuts. Blend until the mushrooms and walnuts are fully incorporated. Set aside.

4.   Place the empty pot over medium-high heat and combine the garlic, celery, and 1 thyme sprig. Sauté for 1 minute.

5.   Add the mushrooms and then the flour. Stir to coat the mushrooms.

6.   Pour in the blended stock and add the milk, wild and brown rice, rosemary sprig, and remaining 2 thyme sprigs. Bring to simmer and cook for half an hour.

7.   Season with pepper and a drizzle of vinegar.

Nutrition Per Serving:

calories: 337 | fat: 12g | carbs: 51g | protein: 12g | fiber: 6g

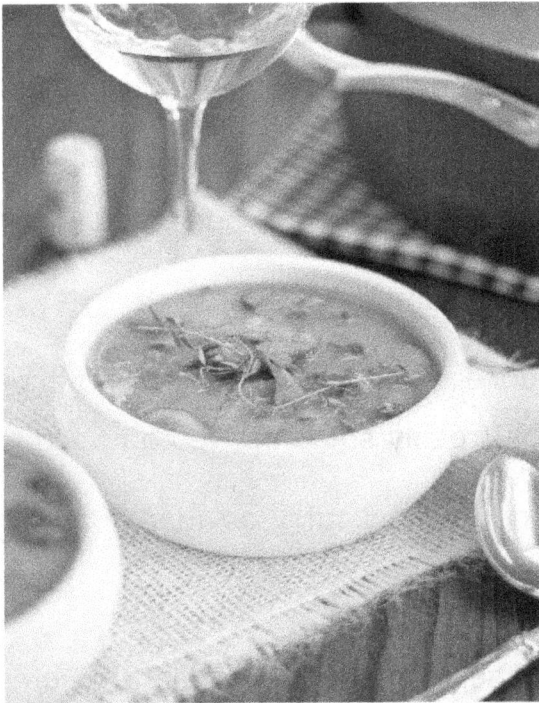

Ginger Carrot Cauliflower Soup

Preparation time: 15 minutes

Cook time: 55 minutes

Serves 6

Ingredients:

6 carrots, coarsely chopped

1 cauliflower head, cut into florets 1 sweet potato, peeled and chopped 1 yellow onion, coarsely chopped 2 garlic cloves, minced

1 tablespoon water, plus more as needed

1 tbsp ginger 1 tsp red pepper flakes

6 cups no-sodium vegetable broth

1 (14-ounce / 397-g) can full-fat coconut milk 1 tablespoon freshly squeezed lemon juice

1 tablespoon yellow curry powder

2 teaspoons ground turmeric

½ cup coarsely chopped fresh cilantro Pumpkin seeds, for serving

Cayenne pepper, for seasoning

Directions:

1. Heat up to 240°C. Line a baking sheet with parchment paper.

2. Spread the carrots, cauliflower, and sweet potato evenly on the prepared baking sheet.

3. Bake for 30 minutes. Flip the vegetables and bake for 10 minutes more, until lightly browned and fork-tender.

4. Put together onion and garlic. Sauté for 2 to 3 minutes. Add the ginger and red pepper flakes and cook for 1 minute more.

5. Bring soup to a boil.

6. Add the roasted vegetables and bring the soup to simmer. Cook for 5 minutes.

7. Add coconut milk, lemon juice, curry powder, and turmeric. Using an immersion blender, purée until smooth. Stir in the cilantro.

8. Garnish with pumpkin seeds and cayenne pepper.

Tomato Gazpacho

Preparation Time: 30 minutes

Cooking Time: 55 minutes

Servings: 6

Ingredients:

1 Tablespoon + 1 Teaspoon Red Wine Vinegar, Divided

½ Teaspoon Pepper 1 Teaspoon Sea Salt 1 Avocado,

¼ Cup Basil, Fresh & Chopped

2 Tablespoons + 2 Teaspoons Olive Oil, Divided 1 Clove Garlic, crushed

1 Red Bell Pepper, Sliced & Seeded 1 Cucumber, Chunked

2 ½ lbs. Large Tomatoes, Cored & Chopped

Directions:

1.   Place half of your cucumber, bell pepper, and ¼ cup of each tomato in a bowl, covering. Set it in the fried.

2.   Puree your remaining tomatoes, cucumber, and bell pepper with garlic, three tablespoons oil, two

tablespoons of vinegar, sea salt, and black pepper into a blender, blending until smooth. Transfer it to a bowl, and chill for two hours.

3. Chop the avocado, adding it to your chopped vegetables, adding your remaining oil, vinegar, salt, pepper, and basil.

4. Ladle your tomato puree mixture into bowls, and serve with chopped vegetables as a salad.

Nutrition:

Calories: 201 Protein: 23g Fat: 4g Carbs: 2g

Cauliflower Asparagus Soup

Preparation Time: 10 minutes

Cooking Time: 30 minutes

Servings: 4

Ingredients:

20 asparagus spears, chopped

4 cups vegetable stock

½ cauliflower head, chopped 2 garlic cloves, chopped

1 tbsp coconut oil Pepper

Salt

Directions:

1.   Heat coconut oil in a saucepan.

2.   Add garlic and sauté until softened.

3.   Add cauliflower, vegetable stock, pepper, and salt. Stir well and bring to boil.

4.   Simmer for 25 minutes.

5.   Add chopped asparagus and cook until softened.

6.   Puree the soup until smooth and creamy.

7.   Stir well and serve warm.

Nutrition:

Calories: 298 Carbs: 26g Protein: 21g Fat: 9g

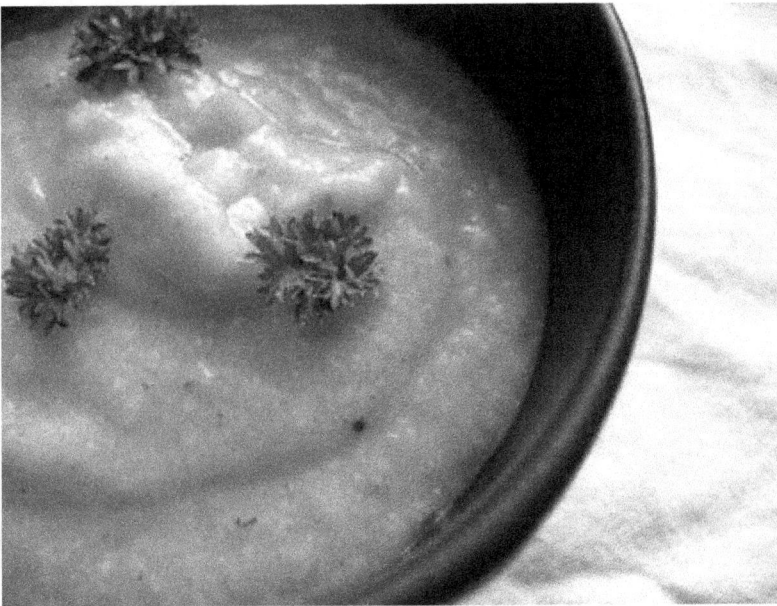

African Pineapple Peanut Stew

Preparation Time: 10 minutes

Cooking Time: 20 minutes

Servings: 4

Ingredients:

4 cups sliced kale

1 cup chopped onion 1/2 cup peanut butter

1 tbsp. Hot pepper sauce or 1 tbsp. Tabasco sauce 2 minced garlic cloves

1/2 cup chopped cilantro

2 cups pineapple, undrained, canned & crushed 1 tbsp. vegetable oil

Directions:

1.   In a saucepan (preferably covered), sauté the garlic and onions in the oil until the onions are lightly browned, approximately 10 minutes, stirring often.

2.   Wash the kale till the time the onions are sautéed.

3.   Get rid of the stems. Mound the leaves on a cutting surface & slice crosswise into slices (preferably 1" thick).

4.   Now, put the pineapple and juice on the onions & bring to a simmer. Stir the kale in, cover, and simmer until just tender, frequently stirring, approximately 5 minutes.

5.   Mix in the hot pepper sauce, peanut butter & simmer for more 5 minutes.

6.   Add salt according to your taste.

Nutrition:

Calories: 402 Carbs: 7g Protein: 21g Fat: 34g

Cabbage & Beet Stew

Preparation Time: 20 minutes

Cooking Time: 10 minutes

Servings: 4

Ingredients:

2 Tablespoons Olive Oil 3 Cups Vegetable Broth

2 Tablespoons Lemon Juice, Fresh

½ Teaspoon Garlic Powder

½ Cup Carrots, Shredded 2 Cups Cabbage, Shredded 1 Cup Beets, Shredded Dill for Garnish

½ Teaspoon Onion Powder

Sea Salt & Black Pepper to Taste

Directions:

1.   Heat oil in a pot, and then sauté your vegetables.

2.   Pour your broth in, mixing in your seasoning. Simmer until it's cooked through, and then top with dill.

Basil Tomato Soup

Preparation Time: 10 minutes

Cooking Time: 10 minutes

Servings: 6

Ingredients:

28 oz. can tomatoes

¼ cup basil pesto

¼ tsp dried basil leaves 1 tsp apple cider vinegar 2 tbsp erythritol

¼ tsp garlic powder

½ tsp onion powder 2 cups water

1 ½ tsp kosher salt

Directions:

1. Add tomatoes, garlic powder, onion powder, water, and salt in a saucepan.

2. Bring to boil over medium heat. Reduce heat and simmer for 2 minutes.

3.   Remove the saucepan from heat and puree the soup using a blender until smooth.

4.   Stir in pesto, dried basil, vinegar, and erythritol.

5.   Stir well and serve warm.

Nutrition:

Calories: 662 Carbs: 18g Protein: 8g Fat: 55g

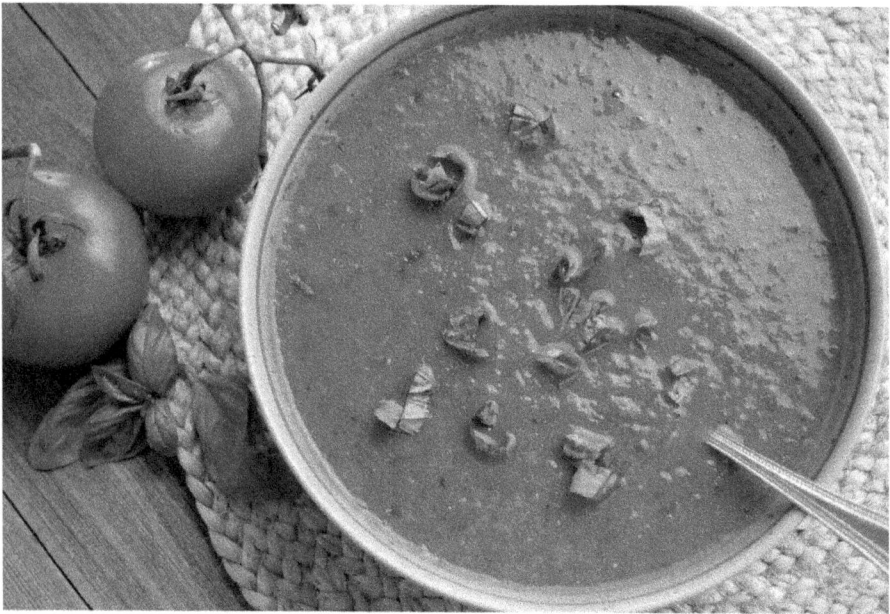

Mushroom & Broccoli Soup

Preparation Time: 20 minutes

Cooking Time: 45 minutes

Servings: 8

Ingredients:

1 bundle broccoli (around 1-1/2 lb.) 1 tablespoon canola oil

1/2 pound cut crisp mushrooms

1 tablespoon diminished sodium soy sauce 2 medium carrots, finely slashed

2 celery ribs, finely slashed 1/4 cup slashed onion 1 garlic clove, minced

1 container (32 oz.) vegetable juices 2 cups of water

2 tablespoons lemon juice

Directions:

1. Cut broccoli florets into reduced down pieces. Strip and hack stalks.

2.   In an enormous pot, heat oil over medium-high warmth; saute mushrooms until delicate, 4-6 minutes. Mix in soy sauce; expel from skillet.

3.   In the same container, join broccoli stalks, carrots, celery, onion, garlic, soup, and water; heat to the point of boiling. Diminish heat; stew, revealed, until vegetables are relaxed, 25-30 minutes.

4.   Puree soup utilizing a drenching blender. Or then again, cool marginally, puree the soup in a blender, come back to the dish.

5.   Mix in florets and mushrooms; heat to the point of boiling. Lessen warmth to medium; cook until broccoli is delicate, 8-10 minutes, blending infrequently. Mix in lemon juice.

Nutrition:

Calories: 830 Carbs: 8g Protein: 45g Fat: 64g

Creamy Cauliflower Pakora Soup

Preparation Time: 20 minutes

Cooking Time: 20 minutes

Servings: 8

Ingredients:

1 giant head cauliflower, cut into little florets 5 medium potatoes, stripped and diced

1 giant onion, diced

4 medium carrots, stripped and diced 2 celery ribs, diced

1 container (32 oz.) vegetable stock 1 teaspoon garam masala

1 teaspoon garlic powder

1 teaspoon ground coriander 1 teaspoon ground turmeric 1 teaspoon ground cumin

1 teaspoon pepper

1 teaspoon salt

1/2 teaspoon squashed red pepper chips Water or extra vegetable stock

New cilantro leaves

Lime wedges, discretionary

Directions:

1.   In a Dutch stove over medium-high warmth, heat initial 14 fixings to the point of boiling. Cook and mix until vegetables are delicate, around 20 minutes. Expel from heat; cool marginally. Procedure in groups in a blender or nourishment processor until smooth. Modify consistency as wanted with water (or extra stock). Sprinkle with new cilantro. Serve hot, with lime wedges whenever wanted.

2.   Stop alternative: Before including cilantro, solidify cooled soup in cooler compartments. To utilize, in part, defrost in cooler medium-term.

3.   Warmth through in a pan, blending every so often and including a little water if fundamental. Sprinkle with cilantro. Whenever wanted, present with lime wedges.

Nutrition:

Calories: 248 Carbs: 7g Protein: 1g Fat: 19g

Garden Vegetable and Herb Soup

Preparation Time: 20 minutes

Cooking Time: 30 minutes

Servings: 8

Ingredients:

2 tablespoons olive oil

2 medium onions, hacked 2 giant carrots, cut

1 pound red potatoes (around 3 medium), cubed 2 cups of water

1 can (14-1/2 oz.) diced tomatoes in sauce 1-1/2 cups vegetable soup

2 tsp garlic powder 1 tsp basil

1/2 tsp salt

1/2 tsp paprika 1/4 tsp weed 1/4 tsp pepper

1 squash 1 zucchini

Directions:

1.   In a huge pan, heat oil over medium warmth. Include onions and carrots; cook and mix until onions are delicate, 4-6 minutes. Include potatoes and cook for 2 minutes. Mix in water, tomatoes, juices, and seasonings.

2.   Heat to the point of boiling. Diminish heat; stew, revealed, until potatoes and carrots are delicate, 9 minutes.

3.   Include yellow squash and zucchini; cook until vegetables are delicate, 9 minutes longer. Serve or, whenever wanted, puree blend in clusters, including extra stock until desired consistency is accomplished.

Nutrition:

Calories: 252 Carbs: 12g Protein: 1g Fat: 11g

Low-Fat Bean Soup

Cook time: 10 minutes

Servings: 4

Ingredients:

2 cans beans

½ cup of salsa

16 oz. vegetable broth

1 tablespoon chili powder

Directions:

1.   Pulse 1 can of beans until almost smooth.

2.   Pour the mixture into a saucepan. Add the remaining can beans, vegetable broth, salsa, and chili powder into the pan.

3. After boil, serve and enjoy!

Protein-Rich Vegetable Minestrone

Preparation time: 30 minutes

Servings: 6

Ingredients:

¼ cup white quinoa, uncooked 1 can (28 oz.) tomatoes, diced 1 cup carrots, sliced

1 ½ cups asparagus, chopped 1 cup packed kale, chopped

½ cup frozen peas

2 cup zucchini chopped 2 bay leaves
1 tablespoon olive oil 4 cups of water

1small white onion, diced 3 garlic cloves, minced

2 teaspoons Italian seasoning Pepper and salt, to taste

Directions:

1. Sauté onions, garlic, and carrots in olive oil over medium-high heat for 3 minutes. Stir in water, tomatoes, quinoa, bay leaves, spices, pepper, and salt, and bring to a boil. Cover and simmer for 20 minutes.

2. Add the remaining vegetable and cook for 10 minutes. Serve hot.

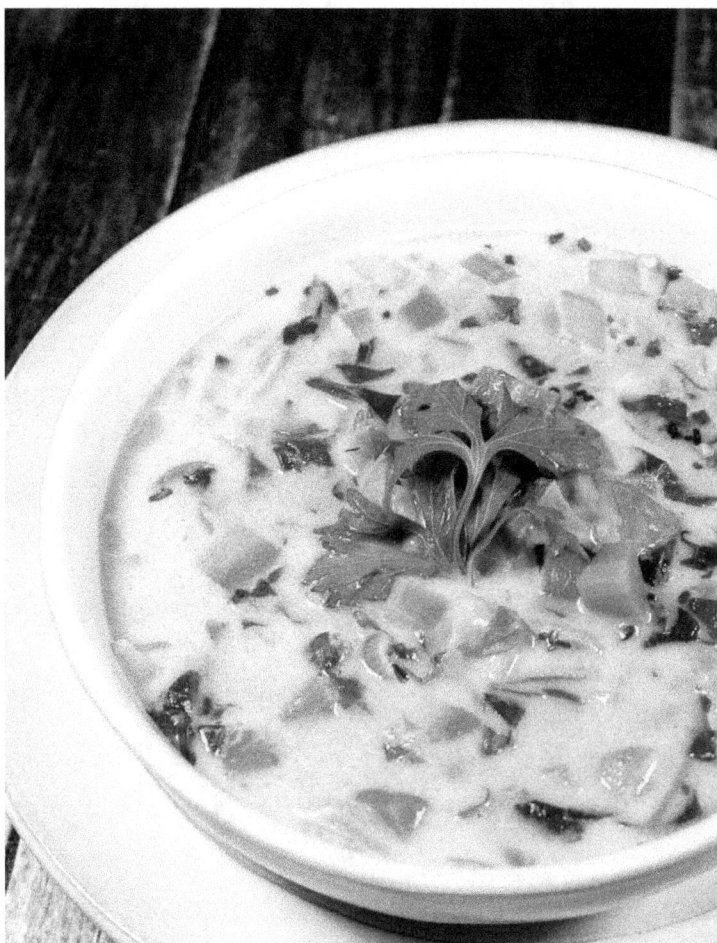

Quinoa Pumpkin Soup

Cook time: 25 minutes

Servings: 4

Ingredients:

½ cup quinoa

20 oz. can black beans, rinsed, drained 3 cups pumpkin, cubed

2 bay leaves

5 cups vegetable broth 1 tablespoon olive oil 1 onion, diced

5 garlic cloves, diced

1 red chili pepper, diced

½ teaspoon dried oregano 1 teaspoon ground cumin

½ teaspoon red pepper flakes, crushed

Directions:

1.   Sauté onions in olive oil over medium until translucent. Stir in red chili pepper and garlic and sauté until aromatic. Mix in the pumpkin and spices and cook for a few minutes.

2.   Pour in quinoa and 2 cups vegetable broth, then bring to a boil. Cook for extra 5 minutes, then add the remaining vegetable broth and cook until boiled. Stir in beans and bay leaves. Simmer for 10 minutes. Serve with avocados.

Tomato Pumpkin Soup

Preparation Time: 25 minutes

Cooking Time: 25 minutes

Servings: 4

Ingredients:

2 cups pumpkin, diced 1/2 cup tomato, chopped 1/2 cup onion, chopped 2 tsp curry 1 tsp paprika

2 cups vegetable stock 1 tsp olive oil

1/2 tsp garlic, minced

Directions:

1.   In a saucepan, add oil, garlic, and onion and sauté for 3 minutes over medium heat.

2.   Add remaining ingredients into the saucepan and bring to boil.

3.   Reduce heat and cover, and simmer for 10 minutes.

4. Puree the soup.

5. Stir well and serve warm.

Nutrition:

Calories: 340 Protein: 50g Carbs: 14g Fat: 10g

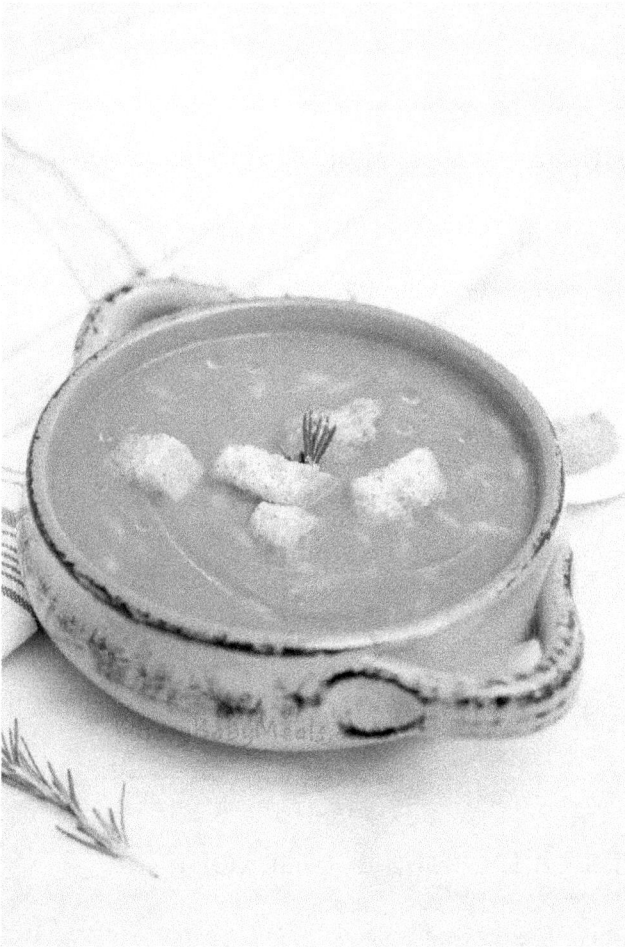

Creamy Garlic Onion Soup

Preparation Time: 45 minutes

Cooking Time: 25 minutes

Servings: 4

Ingredients:

1 onion, sliced

4 cups vegetable stock 1 1/2 tbsp olive oil

1 shallot, sliced

2 garlic clove, chopped

1 leek, sliced Salt

Directions:

1.   Add stock and olive oil in a saucepan and bring to boil.

2.   Add remaining ingredients and stir well.

3.   Cover and simmer for 25 minutes.

4.   Puree the soup until smooth.

5.   Stir well and serve warm.

Avocado Broccoli Soup

Preparation Time: 20 minutes Cooking Time: 5 minutes

Servings: 4

Ingredients:

2 cups broccoli florets, chopped 5 cups vegetable broth

2 avocados, chopped Pepper

Salt

Directions:

1. Cook broccoli for 10 minutes.

2. Add broccoli, vegetable broth, avocados, pepper, and salt to the blender and blend until smooth.

3. Stir well and serve warm.

Nutrition: Calories: 265 Protein: 35g Fat: 13 Carbs: 5

Green Spinach Kale Soup

Preparation Time: 10 minutes

Cooking Time: 5 minutes

Servings: 6

Ingredients:

2 avocados

8 oz. spinach

8 oz. kale

1 fresh lime juice 1 cup water

3 1/3 cup coconut milk 3 oz. olive oil

1/4 tsp pepper 1 tsp salt

Directions:

1.   Heat the oil in a saucepan.

2.   Add kale and spinach to the saucepan and sauté for 2-3 minutes. Remove saucepan from heat. Add coconut milk, spices, avocado, and water. Stir well.

3.   Puree the soup until smooth and creamy. Add fresh lime juice and stir well.

4.   Serve and enjoy.

Nutrition:

Calories: 312 Protein: 9g Fat: 10 Carbs: 22

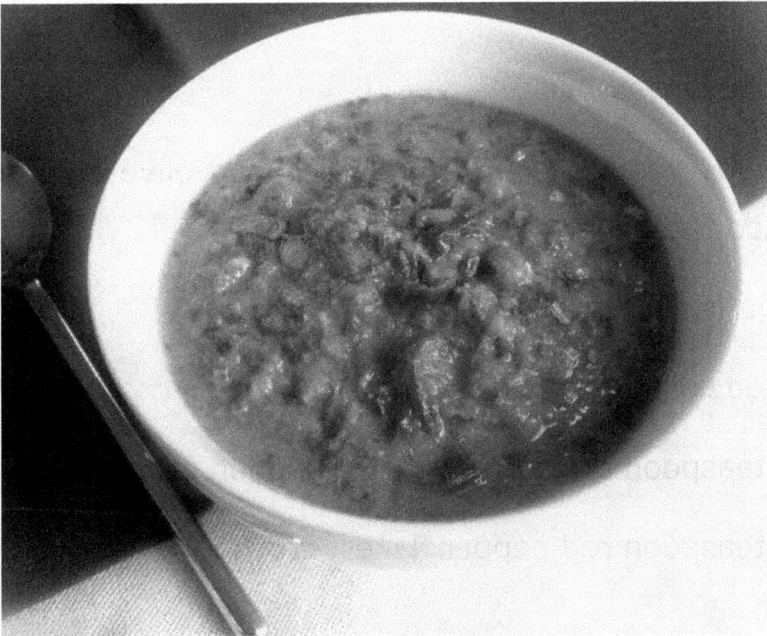

Quinoa Pumpkin Soup

Cook time: 25 minutes

Servings: 4

Ingredients:

½ cup quinoa

20 oz. can black beans, rinsed, drained 3 cups pumpkin, cubed

2 bay leaves

5 cups vegetable broth 1 tablespoon olive oil 1 onion, diced

5 garlic cloves, diced

1 red chili pepper, diced

½ teaspoon dried oregano 1 teaspoon ground cumin

½ teaspoon red pepper flakes, crushed

Directions:

1.   Sauté onions in olive oil over medium until translucent. Stir in red chili pepper and garlic and sauté until aromatic. Mix in the pumpkin and spices and cook for a few minutes.

2.   Pour in quinoa and 2 cups vegetable broth, then bring to a boil. Cook for extra 5 minutes, then add the remaining vegetable broth and cook until boiled. Stir in beans and bay leaves. Simmer for 10 minutes. Serve with avocados.

Incredible Tomato Basil Soup

Total time: 6 hours 10 minutes

Ingredients:

1 cup celery 1 cup carrots

74 ounces of whole tomatoes, canned 2 cups of chopped white onion

2 tsp garlic 1 tbsp of salt

1/2 teaspoon of ground white pepper

1/4 cup of basil leaves and more for garnishing 1 bay leaf

32 fluid ounce of vegetable broth 1/2 cup of grated Parmesan cheese

Directions:

1.   Using 8 quarts or a larger slow cooker, place all the ingredients.

2.   Stir until it mixes properly and covers the top.

3.   Plug in the slow cooker; adjust the cooking time to 5 hours and let it cook on the high heat setting or until the vegetables are tender.

4.   Blend the soup with a submersion blender or until the soup reaches your desired state.

5.   Garnish it with cheese, basil leaves, and serve.

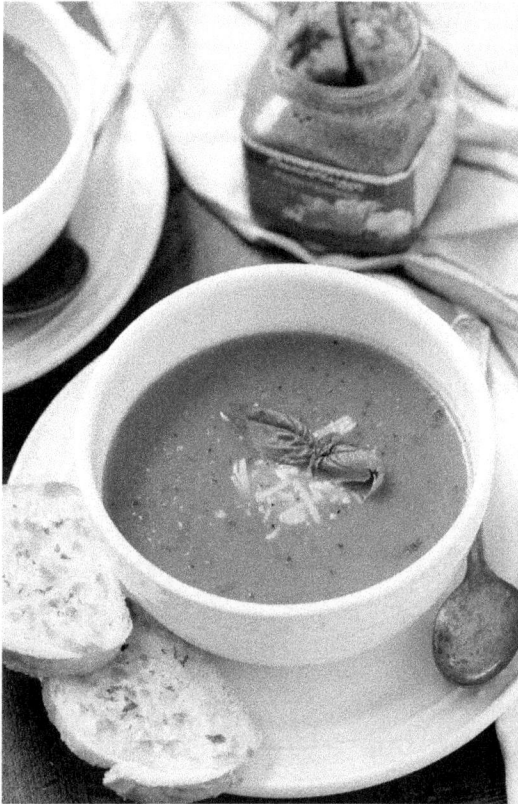

Sizzling Vegetarian Fajitas

Total time: 2 hours 25 minutes

Ingredients:

4 ounces of diced green chilies 3 medium-sized tomatoes, diced

1 large green bell pepper, cored and sliced

2 red peppers, cored and sliced

1 medium-sized white onion, peeled and sliced 1/2 teaspoon of garlic powder

1/4 teaspoon of salt

2 teaspoons of red chili powder 2 teaspoons of ground cumin 1/2 teaspoon of dried oregano 1 1/2 tablespoon of olive oil

Directions:

1.   Take a 6-quart slow cooker, grease it with a non-stick cooking spray and add all the ingredients.

2.   Stir until it mixes properly and covers the top.

3. Plug in the slow cooker; adjust the cooking time to 2 hours and let it cook on the high heat setting or until it cooks thoroughly.

4. Serve with tortillas.

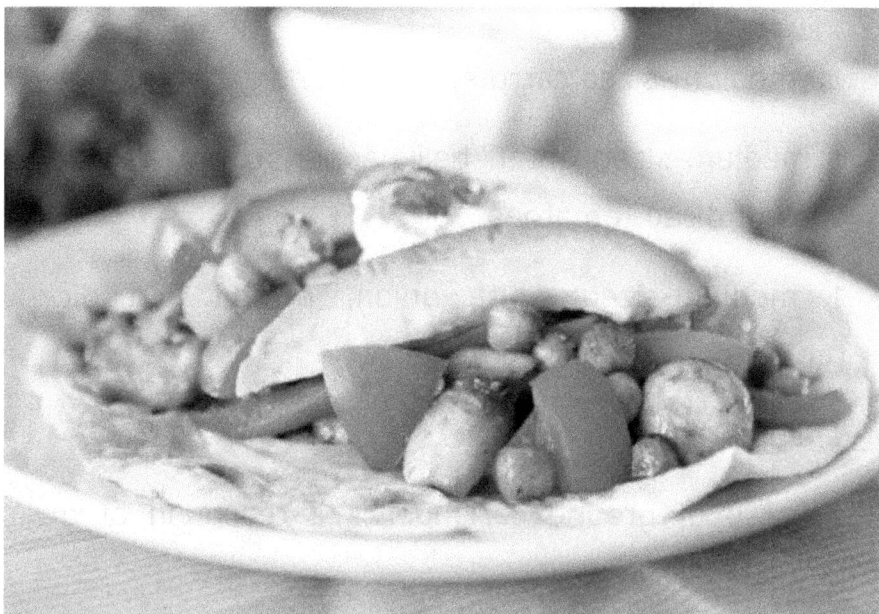

Chunky Black Lentil Veggie Soup

Total time: 4 hours 35 minutes

Ingredients:

1 1/2 cups of black lentils, uncooked 2 small turnips, peeled and diced

10 medium-sized carrots, peeled and diced

1 medium-sized green bell pepper, cored and diced 3 cups of diced tomatoes

1 medium-sized white onion, peeled and diced 2 tablespoons of minced ginger

1 tsp garlic 1 tsp of salt

1/2 tsp of ground coriander 1/2 teaspoon of ground cumin

3 tablespoons of unsalted butter 32 fluid ounce of vegetable broth 32 fluid ounces of water

Directions:

1.   Using a medium-sized microwave, cover the bowl, place the lentils, and pour in the water.

2.   Microwave lentils for 10 minutes or until softened, stirring after 5 minutes.

3.   Drain lentils and add to a 6-quart slow cooker and remaining ingredients and stir until just mix.

4.   Cover with top, plugin slow cooker; adjust cooking time to 6 hours, and cook on low heat setting or until carrots are tender.

5.   Serve straight away.

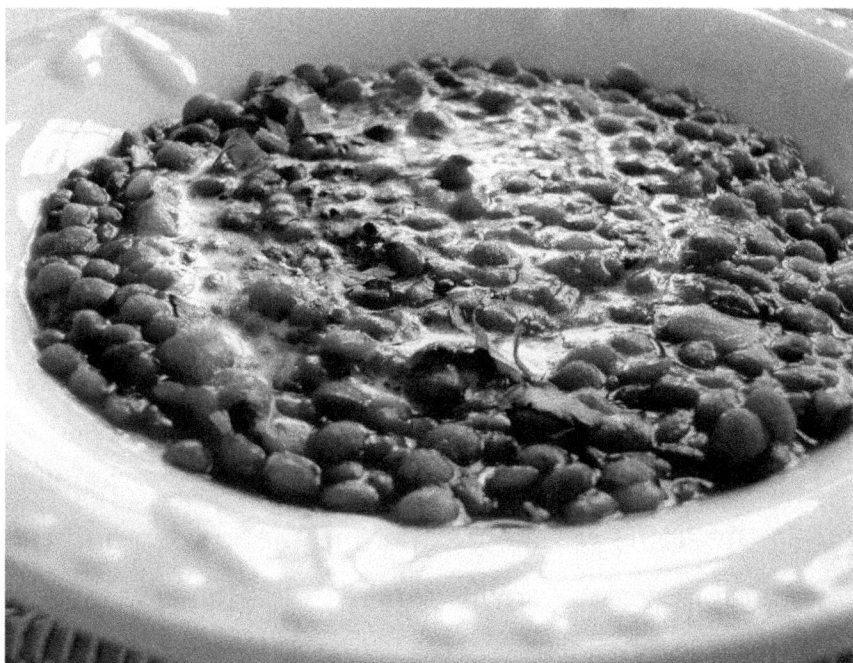

Creamy Artichoke Soup

Preparation Time: 5 minutes

Cooking Time: 40 minutes

Servings: 4

Ingredients:

1 can artichoke hearts, drained 3 cups vegetable broth

2 tbsp. lemon juice

1 small onion, finely cut 2 cloves garlic, crushed 3 tbsp. olive oil

2 tbsp. flour

½ cup vegan cream

Directions:

1.   Gently sauté the onion and garlic in some olive oil. Add the flour, whisking constantly, and then add the hot vegetable broth slowly while still whisking. Cook for about 5 minutes.

2.   Blend the artichoke, lemon juice, salt, and pepper until smooth. Add the puree to the broth mix, stir well, and then stir in the cream. Cook until heated through. Garnish with a swirl of vegan cream or a sliver of artichoke.

Nutrition:

Calories: 1622 kcal Protein: 4.45 g Fat: 181.08 g Carbohydrates: 10.99 g

Italian Herb Squash Soup

Preparation time: 17 minutes

Cook time: 35 minutes

Serves 4

Ingredients:

3 cups butternut squash

1 potato

1 onion (about ½ cup) 1 clove garlic, peeled and chopped

¼ tsp dried Italian herb mix

¼ cup green peas

¼ teaspoon fresh lime juice Finely chopped parsley

Directions:

1.   Bring a large pot to boil. Add the squash, potato, onion, garlic, herb mix, and pepper. Cook until the vegetables are tender.

2.   Purée the soup using an immersion blender or in a blender with a tight-fitting lid, covered with a towel. Put

in the pot the green peas and lime juice. Cook for an additional 5 to 7 minutes, or until the peas are tender. Serve hot, garnished with parsley.

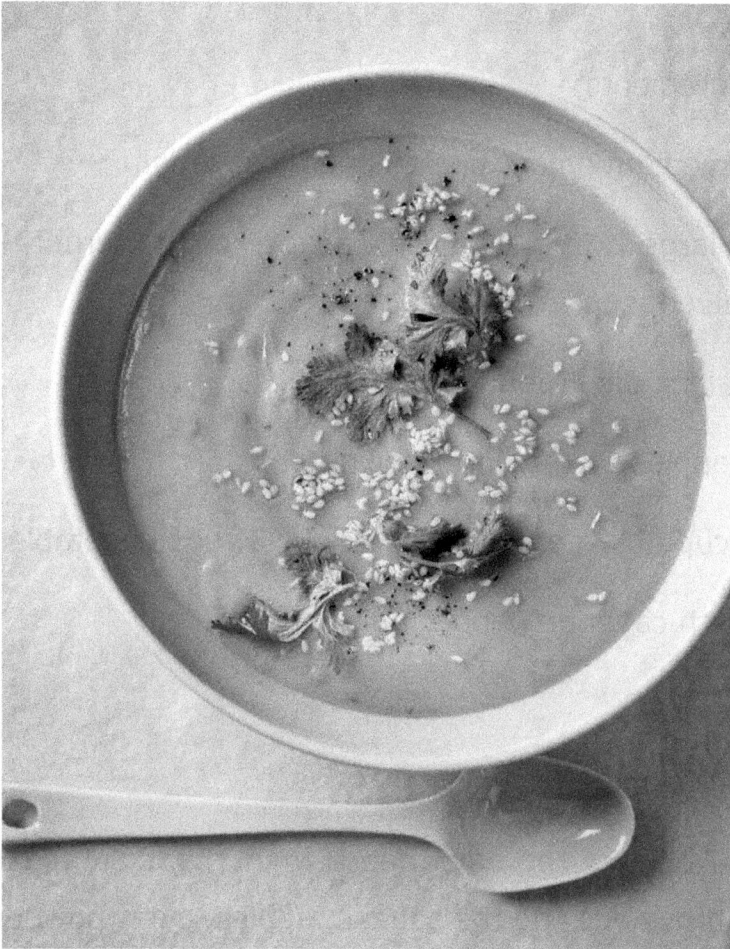

Curried Winter Squash and Apple Soup

Preparation time: 15 minutes

Cook time: 35 minutes

Serves 4

Ingredients:

1 medium onion, peeled and diced small

1 large winter squash, acorn, or butternut, peeled, halved, seeded, and cut into

½-inch dice (about 6 cups)

2 apples 1 tbsp curry powder

1 cup unsweetened apple cider 3 cups vegetable stock

Pinch cayenne pepper Salt to taste

Directions:

1.   Sauté the onion for 10 minutes, or until the onion is browned. Add the squash, apples, curry powder, cider, vegetable stock, and cayenne pepper, and bring to a boil over high heat.

2.   Cook for about 20 minutes or until the squash is tender. Purée the soup using an immersion blender or in batches in a blender with a tight-fitting lid, covered with a towel. Season with salt.

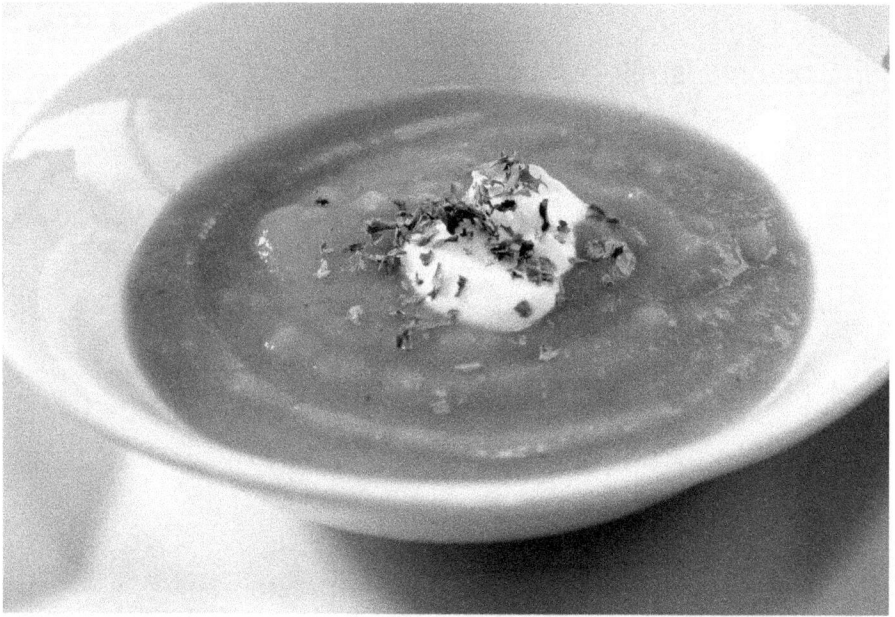

Chestnut Soup with Carrot

Preparation time: 10 minutes

Cook time: 25 minutes

Serves 4

Ingredients:

1 onion 1 stalk celery

1 carrot 1½ tbsp sage

1 tbsp thyme 1 bay leaf

⅛ tsp ground cloves 5 cups vegetable stock

1 (15-ounce /425-g) can chestnut purée

Salt and black pepper 2 tbsp parsley

Directions:

1.   Sauté the onion, celery and carrot for 15 minutes. Add the sage, thyme, bay leaf, cloves, and vegetable stock. Bring the pot to a boil over high heat and whisk in the chestnut purée. Season and finish cooking for 5 minutes.

Serve garnished with the chopped parsley.

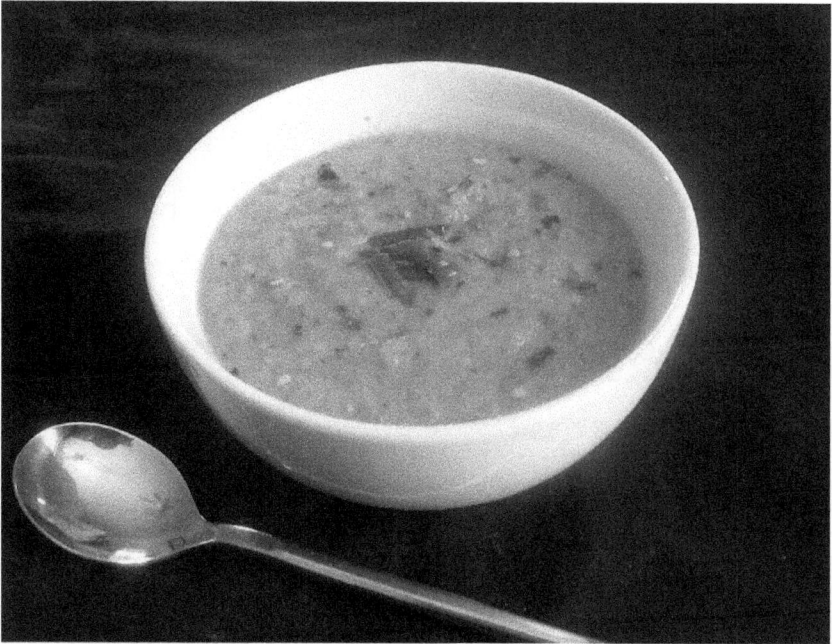

Garlic White Bean and Mushroom Stew

Preparation time: 10 minutes

Cook time: 28 minutes

Serves 4

Ingredients:

1 medium onion, peeled and diced

1 pound (454 g) cremini mushrooms, halved 6 cloves garlic, peeled and chopped

1 (14-ounce / 397-g) can diced tomatoes

¼ cup minced basil

1 tablespoon minced thyme

2 teaspoons minced rosemary 1 bay leaf

4 cups cooked navy beans, or 2 (15-ounce /425-g) cans, drained and rinsed Salt and freshly ground black pepper, to taste

Directions:

1. Sauté the onion and mushrooms for 10 minutes. Stir in the tomatoes, basil, thyme, rosemary, bay leaf, and beans, and bring the pot to a boil over high heat.

2. Cook for 15 minutes. Season with salt and pepper.

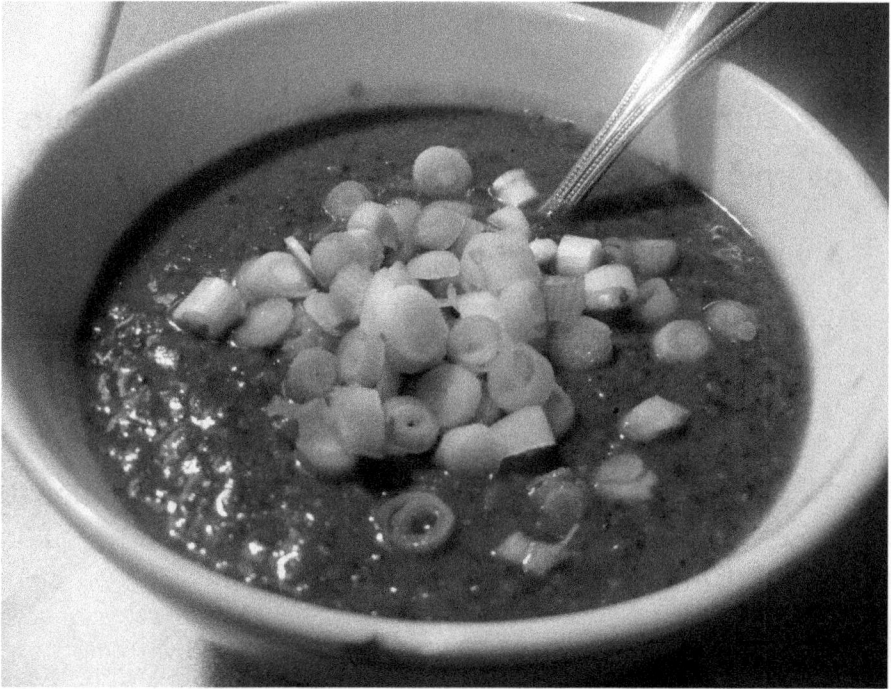

Lima Bean Stew with Carrots

Preparation time: 15 minutes

Cook time: 1¼ hours

Serves 6

Ingredients:

1½ cups dried lima beans, soaked for 8 to 10 hours (or overnight), and drained 2 bay leaves

4 whole cloves

4 cloves garlic, peeled

2 onions 2 celery stalks, chopped

2 carrots 1 green bell pepper 1 teaspoon thyme leaves

¼ cup tomato sauce

Salt and black pepper, to taste

Directions:

1.   Place the soaked lima beans in a pot with 4 cups water and add the bay leaves, cloves, and garlic. Simmer until just tender, adding more water as needed to cover

the beans well. Remove the bay leaves, cloves, and garlic.

2.   Put together onions, celery, and carrots and sauté for 10 minutes. Add the green pepper and thyme and cook for 4 minutes. Add the tomato paste and cook for 1 minute.

3.   Add the vegetable mixture to the cooked beans and cook for 15 minutes over medium heat. Season with salt and pepper.

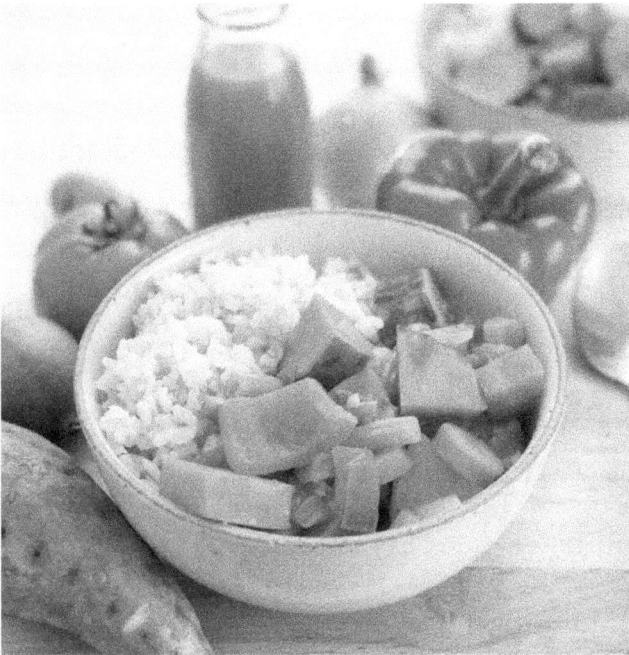

Cilantro Millet Stew

Preparation time: 20 minutes

Cook time: 45 minutes

Serves 4 to 6

Ingredients:

5 to 6 cups vegetable stock

2 (1-inch) pieces cinnamon stick 2 tablespoons grated ginger

1 bay leaf

1 large onion, peeled and cut into ¾-inch pieces 2 large carrots, peeled and cut into ½-inch slices 2 cloves garlic, peeled and minced

1 cup millet

1 large head cauliflower, cut into large florets 1 (14½-ounce / 411-g) can diced tomatoes Salt and freshly ground black pepper, to taste

½ cup chopped cilantro

Directions:

1. In a small pot, combine the vegetable stock, cinnamon sticks, ginger, and bay leaf and cook over medium-high heat for 15 minutes. Remove from the heat, discard the spices, and set the vegetable stock aside.

2. Place the onion and carrots in a large saucepan over medium heat and sauté for 12 minutes. Add the prepared vegetable stock, millet, cauliflower, garlic and tomatoes and take it to boil. Cook until the cauliflower and millet are tender. Season with salt and cook for another 5 minutes.

3. Serve garnished with cilantro.

Quinoa Vegetable Soup

Preparation time: 20 minutes

Cook time: 3 to 8 hours

Serves 6

Ingredients:

1 cup dried quinoa

½ onion 2 garlic cloves

2 carrots, cut into coins

2 celery stalks, cut into slices

1 tablespoon water, plus more as needed

¼ cup tomato paste

1 zucchini, cut into coins, and quartered

1 (14-ounce / 397-g) can whole-kernel corn, drained 1 (14-ounce / 397-g) can diced tomatoes

1 (15-ounce /425-g) black beans, drained and rinsed

1 can red kidney beans 2 tsp chili powder

1 teaspoon ground cumin

6 cups no-sodium vegetable broth, plus more as needed

Directions:

1.   Rinse the quinoa until the cloudy water becomes clear.

2.   On a 5-quart or larger slow cooker, set the temperature to High and let it heat for 5 to 10 minutes.

3.   In the preheated slow cooker, combine the onion, garlic, carrots, celery, and 1 tablespoon of water. Cook for 2 to 3 minutes. Stir in the tomato paste to combine.

4.   Add the zucchini, corn, tomatoes, black beans, kidney beans, chili powder, cumin, and vegetable broth. Stir well. The tomato paste will fully incorporate as the soup cooks.

5.   Turn the heat to low. Cook 6 to 8 hours.

Nutrition Per Serving:

calories: 334 | fat: 4g | carbs: 62g | protein: 16g | fiber: 14g

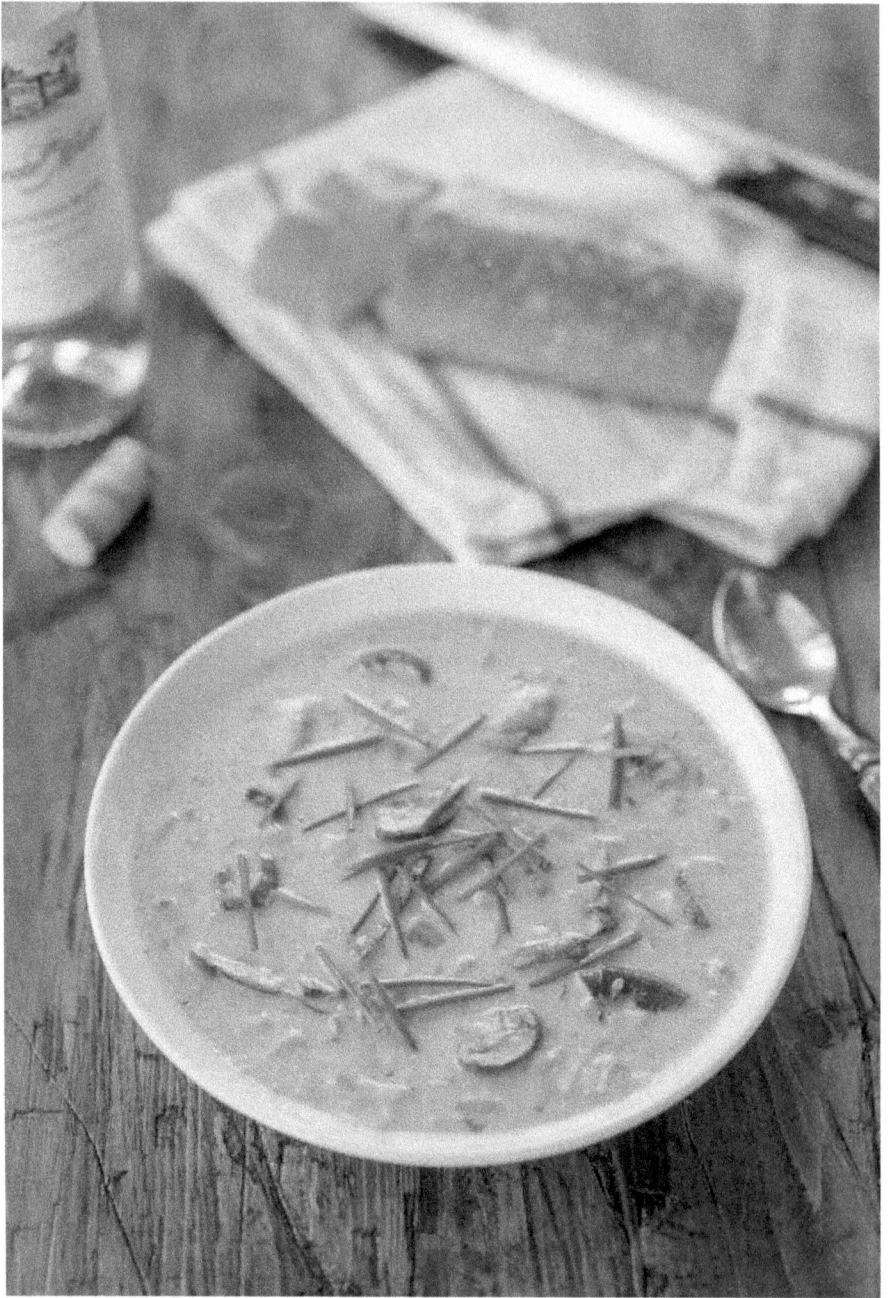

Lemon Asparagus and Leek Soup

Preparation time: 15 minutes

Cook time: 35 minutes

Serves 4

Ingredients:

2 leeks

1 tablespoon water

2 garlic cloves, minced

¾ teaspoon dried tarragon (or dried dill or thyme) 1 cup dried red lentils

1 pound (454 g) asparagus, cut into 1-inch pieces, including the ends 6 cups no-sodium vegetable broth

Juice of 1 lemon

Fresh ground black pepper, to taste

Directions:

1.   Cut off the leeks' root ends and the dark green portion of the stalks. Slit the remaining white and light

green portion lengthwise down the center and run the leeks under cool water, using your fingers to remove any dirt between the layers. Thinly slice the leeks.

2.   Put together the leeks and water. Sauté for 5 minutes. Add the garlic and tarragon. Cook for 2 minutes more.

3.   Add the lentils, asparagus, and vegetable broth. Bring the soup to a boil and cook until the lentils are tender.

4.   Remove some of the cooked lentils, leeks, and asparagus if you'd like some larger pieces in your soup. Purée the soup until slightly chunky. Stir in the ingredients removed if using.

5.   Serve with lemon and pepper.

Nutrition Per Serving:

calories: 243 | fat: 2g | carbs: 45g | protein: 16g | fiber: 8g

Lentil-Miso Kale Soup

Preparation time: 15 minutes

Cook time: 35 minutes

Serves 4

Ingredients:

2 garlic cloves, minced 2 small shallots, diced

4 large carrots, thinly sliced 4 celery stalks, thinly sliced

1 tablespoon water, plus more as needed

3 cups baby potatoes, halved and quartered 4 cups no-sodium vegetable broth

1 tablespoon red miso paste

¼ tsp black pepper 3 thyme sprigs

1 cup lentils 2 cups coarsely chopped kale

Directions:

1. Put together the garlic, shallots, carrots, and celery. Cook for 1 to 2 minutes, adding water, 1

tablespoon at a time, to prevent burning until the shallots and celery start to become translucent.

2.   Add the potatoes and cook for 3 to 4 minutes.

3.   Carefully pour in the vegetable broth. Add the miso paste, pepper, thyme, and lentils. Cook until the lentils and potatoes are tender.

4.   Add the kale and cook for 3 to 4 minutes until wilted.

Nutrition Per Serving:

calories: 292 | fat: 2g | carbs: 58g | protein: 15g | fiber: 12g

Turmeric Chickpea Vegetable Soup

Preparation time: 15 minutes

Cook time: 30 minutes

Serves 4

Ingredients:

1 onion 2 carrots, coarsely chopped

2 celery stalks, coarsely chopped

1 red bell pepper, coarsely chopped 3 garlic cloves, minced

1 tablespoon water, plus more as needed

2 teaspoons grated peeled fresh ginger

1 cauliflower head 1 teaspoon ground turmeric

1 teaspoon Hungarian sweet paprika

6 cups no-sodium vegetable broth 2 cups chopped kale

1 (15-ounce /425-g) can chickpeas, rinsed and drained
Freshly ground black pepper to taste

Chopped scallions, green parts only, for garnish

Directions:

1.   Put together the onion, carrots, celery, bell pepper, and garlic.

2.   Cook adding the ginger and stirring, for 30 seconds.

3.   Stir in the cauliflower, turmeric, and paprika to coat the cauliflower evenly with the spices.

4.   Add the vegetable broth and bring to a simmer. Cook for 10 minutes.

5.   Add the kale and chickpeas and cook for 5 minutes to soften the kale leaves. Season with pepper and garnish with scallions.

Nutrition Per Serving:

calories: 173 | fat: 3g | carbs: 32g | protein: 8g | fiber: 9g

www.ingramcontent.com/pod-product-compliance
Lightning Source LLC
Chambersburg PA
CBHW050759030426
42336CB00012B/1873